It's Catching

Flu

Elizabeth Laskey

Designed by Patricia Stevenson
Printed and bound in the United States by Lake Book Manufacturing

07 06 05 04 03
10 9 8 7 6 5 4 3 2 1

Library of Congress Cataloging-in-Publication Data
Laskey, Elizabeth, 1961–
        Flu / Elizabeth Laskey.
        v. cm. — (It's catching)
        Includes bibliographical references and index.
        Contents: What is flu? — Healthy nose and throat —
        What causes flu? — First signs — Other signs — How flu spreads —
        Treatment — Flu can be dangerous — Flu shots — How flu shots work —
        Flu epidemics — Staying healthy — Think about it.
        ISBN 1-4034-0273-6
        1. Influenza—Juvenile literature. [1. Influenza. 2. Diseases.]
        I. Title. II. Series.

RC150 .L37 2002
616.2'03—dc21
                                        2001008561

Acknowledgments
The author and publishers are grateful to the following for permission to reproduce copyright material:
Cover photograph by Reflections Photolibrary/Corbis
pp. 4, 16 Rob Lewine/Corbis Stock Market; p. 5 Steve Weber/Stock Boston, Inc./PictureQuest; p. 6 Tom and Dee Ann McCarthy/Corbis Stock Market; p. 7 George Shelley/Corbis Stock Market; p. 8 Gopal Murti/PhotoTake; p. 9 PhotoDisc; p. 10 Mary Kate Denny/PhotoEdit/PictureQuest; p. 11 Steve Gottlieb/Stock Connection/PictureQuest; p. 12 Philip James Corwin/Corbis; p. 13 Reporters Press Agency/eStock Photography/PictureQuest; pp. 14, 29 Bob Daemmrich/Stock Boston; p. 15 Reflections Photo Library/Corbis; p. 17 Richard Hutchings/PhotoEdit; p. 18 Bachmann/Photo Researchers, Inc.; p. 19 Tom Stewart/Corbis Stock Market; p. 20 Peter Ardito/Index Stock Imagery/PictureQuest; p. 21 Ronnie Kaufman/Corbis Stock Market; p. 22 Roy Morsch/Corbis Stock Market; p. 23 Richard Hutchings/Photo Researchers, Inc.; pp. 24, 25 Bettmann/Corbis; p. 26 Michael Newman/PhotoEdit; p. 27 David Young-Wolff/PhotoEdit/PictureQuest; p. 28 T. Bannor/Custom Medical Stock Photo.
Every effort has been made to contact copyright holders of any material reproduced in this book. Any omissions will be rectified in subsequent printings if notice is given to the publisher.

Some words are shown in bold, **like this.** You can find out what they mean by looking in the glossary.

Contents

What Is Flu?

Flu is a sickness that makes your body hurt. When you get it, you feel very tired. You may also have a sore throat, a cough, and a runny or stuffy nose.

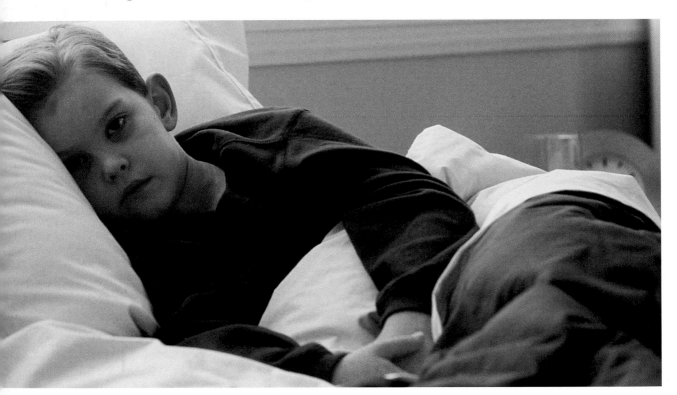

Flu is an **infectious** illness. This means it can spread from one person to another.

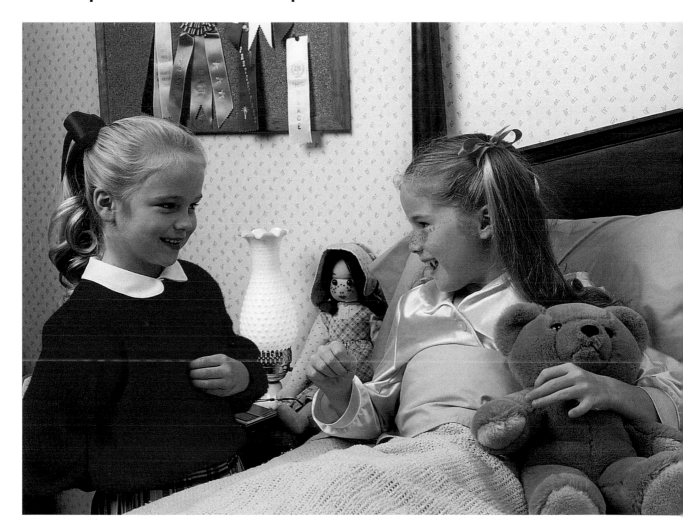

Healthy Nose and Throat

Your nose and throat help keep **germs** from making you sick. Your nose and throat have sticky insides called **mucous membranes.** They trap many germs that get in through your nose and mouth.

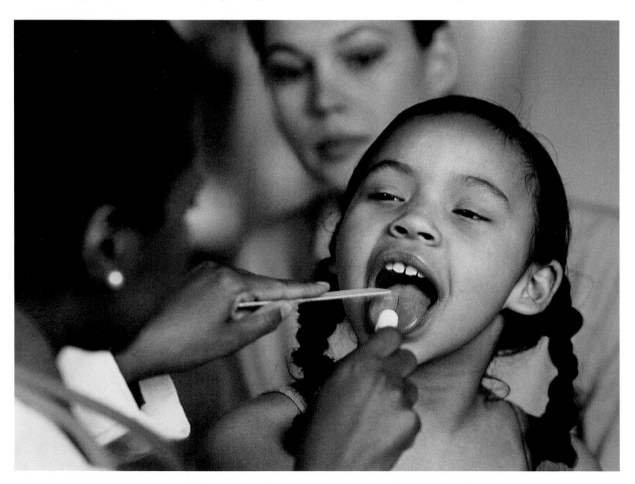

Sneezing and coughing are ways your body tries to get rid of trapped germs. Sneezing and coughing force germs out of your body. This helps keep you from getting sick.

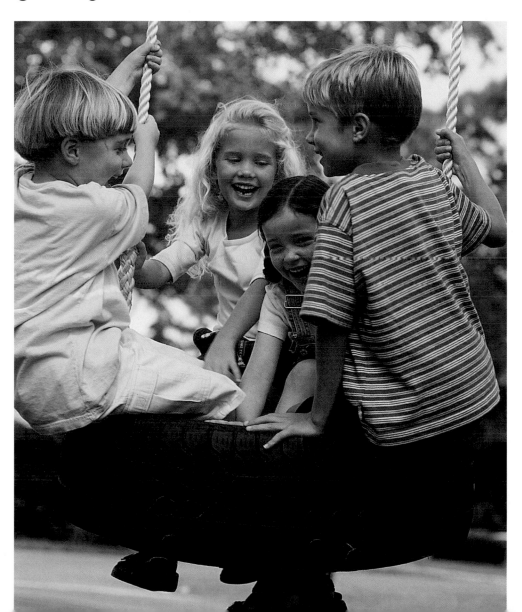

What Causes Flu?

Flu is caused by a **virus,** which is a very tiny **germ.** The flu virus is so small you need a **microscope** to see it. This is what flu viruses look like through a microscope.

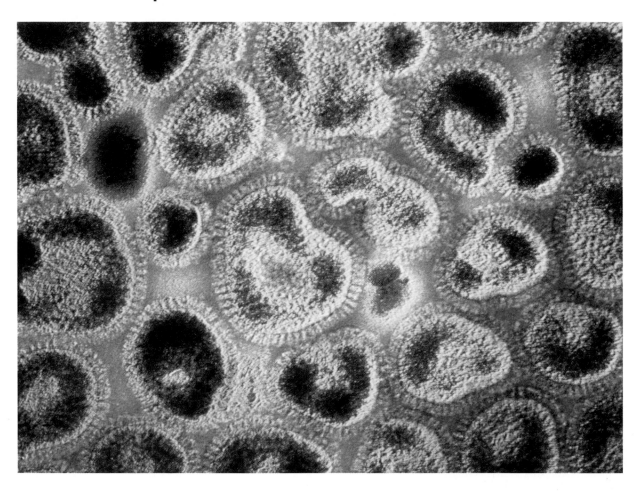

If the virus gets into your body, it can make many more viruses. Then you will get flu. Most people get flu from December to March. This time of year is sometimes called flu season.

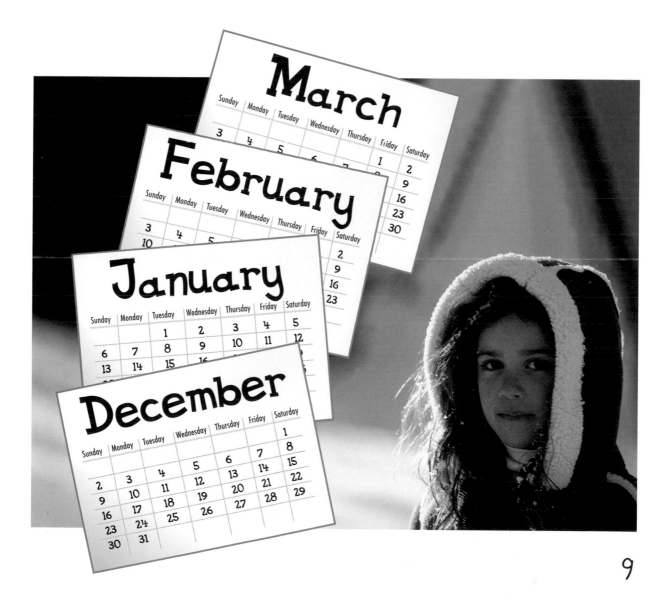

How Flu Spreads

Flu spreads when a person who has flu coughs or sneezes into the air. This sends the flu **virus** into the air. If you breathe in the virus, you may catch flu one to four days later.

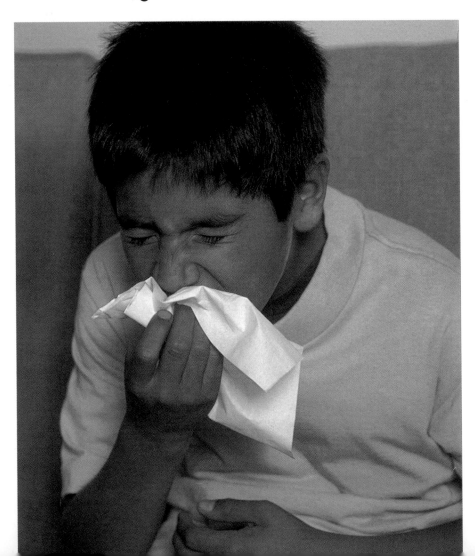

You can spread flu to other people even before you feel the signs of it. When you have flu, you will stay **infectious** for as long as you feel sick.

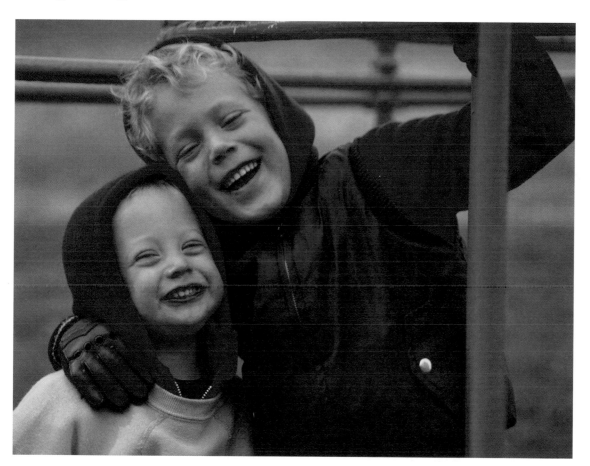

First Signs

When you get flu, your body will start to hurt. Your head may hurt, too. You will probably have a sore throat, a cough, and a **fever.**

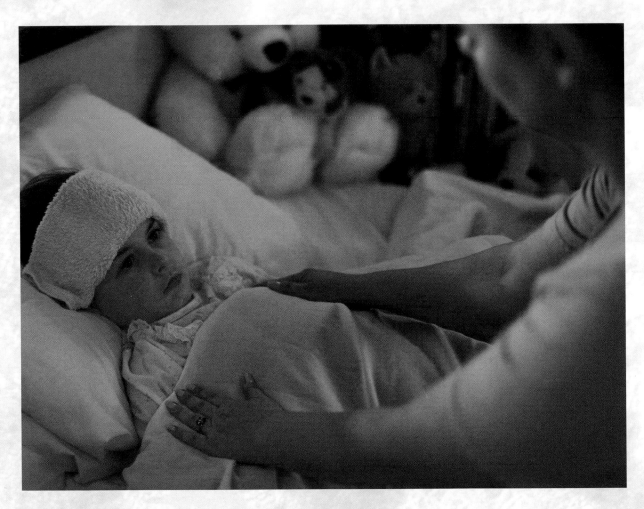

When you have a fever, your body's **temperature** is hotter than normal. A fever is one way your body fights **infection.**

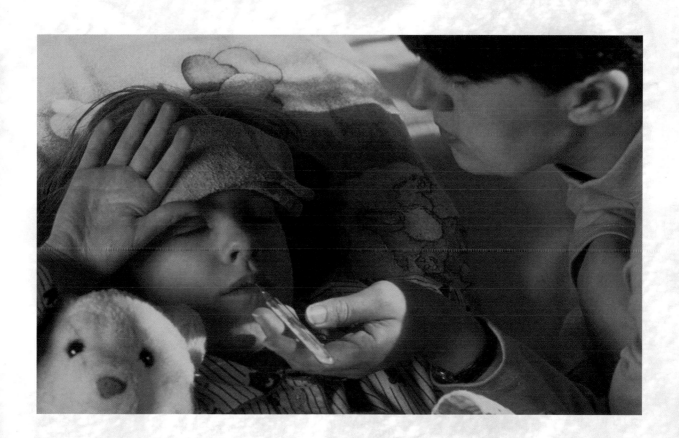

Other Signs

When you have flu, you will feel very tired. You might also feel very cold sometimes. But then a few minutes later you may start to feel very hot.

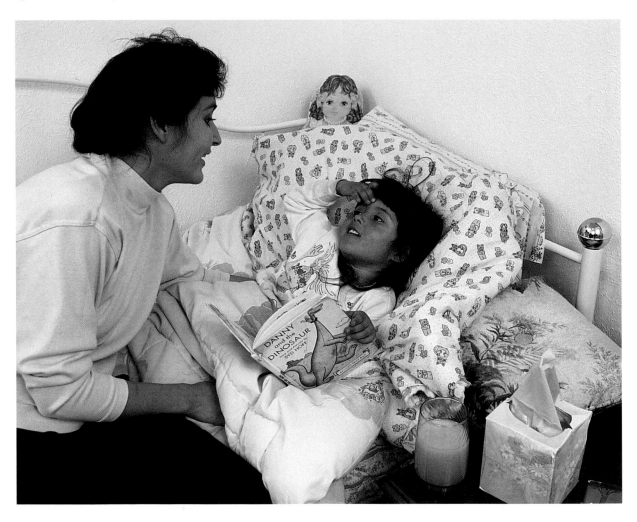

You may also get a stuffy or runny nose.
Some people also get an upset stomach
and do not feel like eating.

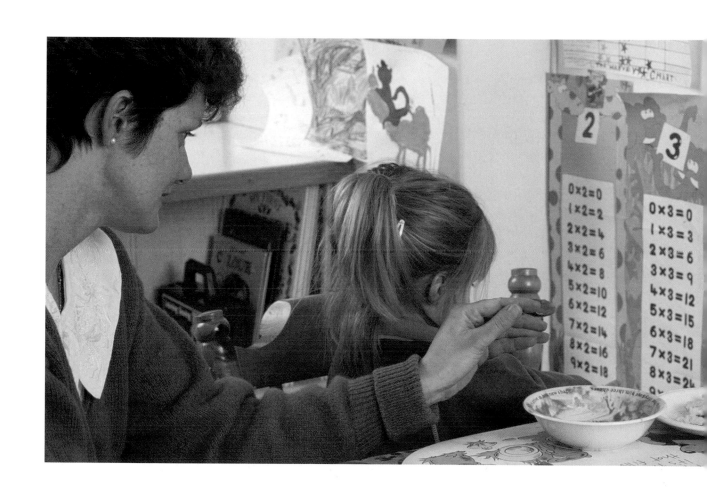

Treatment

If you have flu, you should stay home and rest. Resting lets your body work on getting rid of the **virus.** Drinking lots of water will also help your body get rid of the virus.

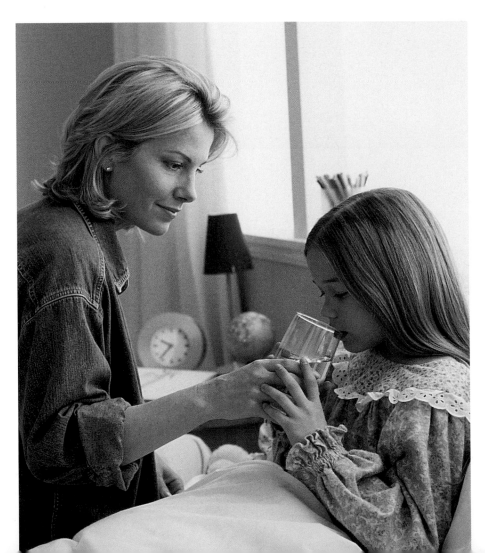

An adult may give you a **pain reliever** to make your head and body hurt less. It will also make your **fever** go down. Most people who get flu feel better in about one week.

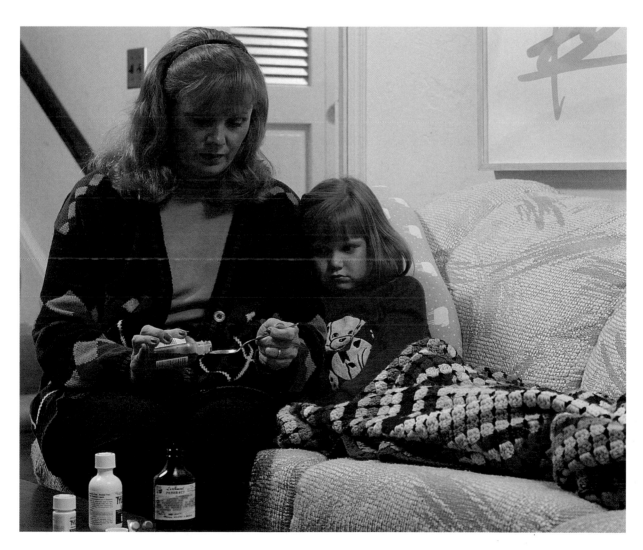

Flu Can Be Dangerous

In older people, flu can sometimes lead to a dangerous **infection** of the **lungs** called **pneumonia.** Younger people with certain health problems may also get lung infections after having flu.

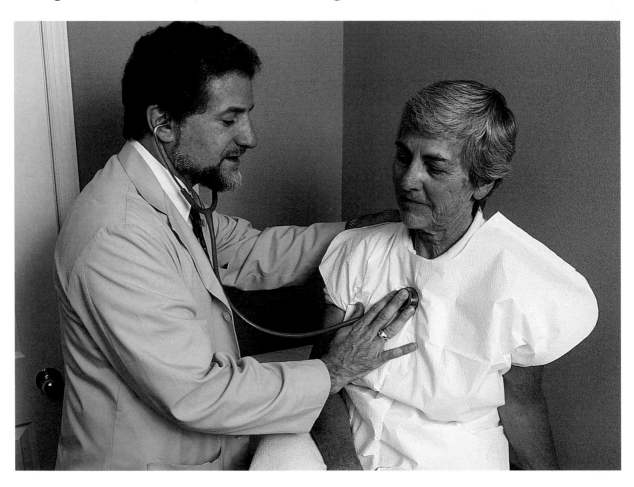

People who get lung infections from flu need to see a doctor. They need medicine to get better. They may also have to go to the hospital.

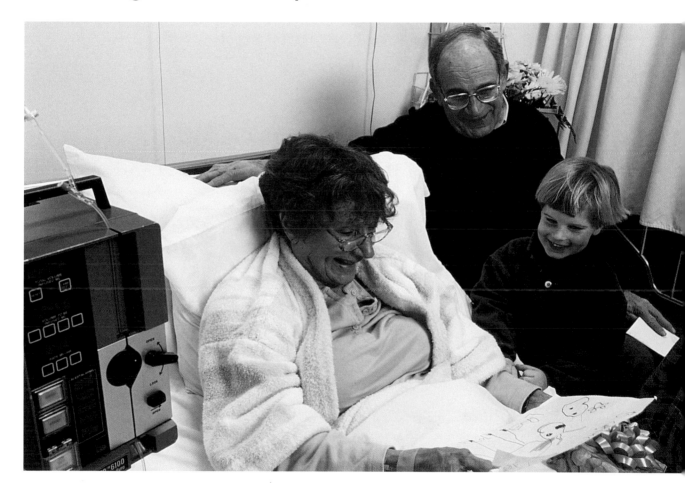

Flu Shots

It is a good idea for older people and younger people with health problems to get a flu shot, or **vaccine.** The flu shot helps keep people from catching flu.

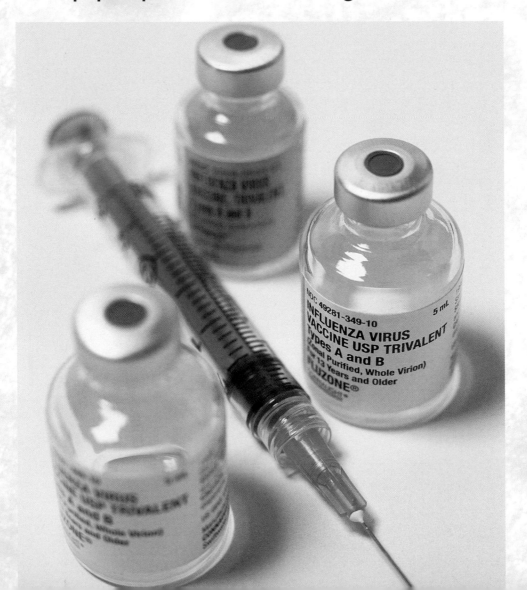

The best time to get a flu shot is from September to November. People get the shot right before flu season starts.

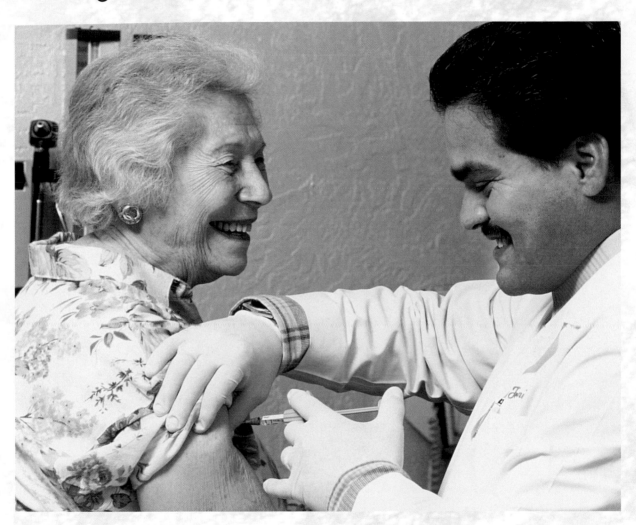

How Flu Shots Work

A flu shot is made from some parts of the flu **virus.** A flu shot helps your body attack the flu virus to keep it from making you sick.

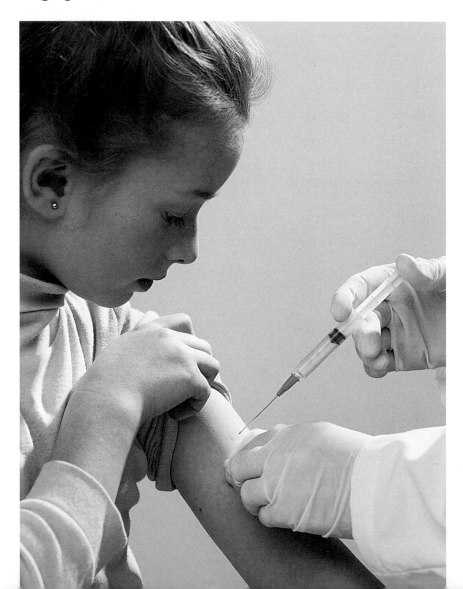

The shot can protect you from getting flu. It will help give you **immunity** to the flu virus.

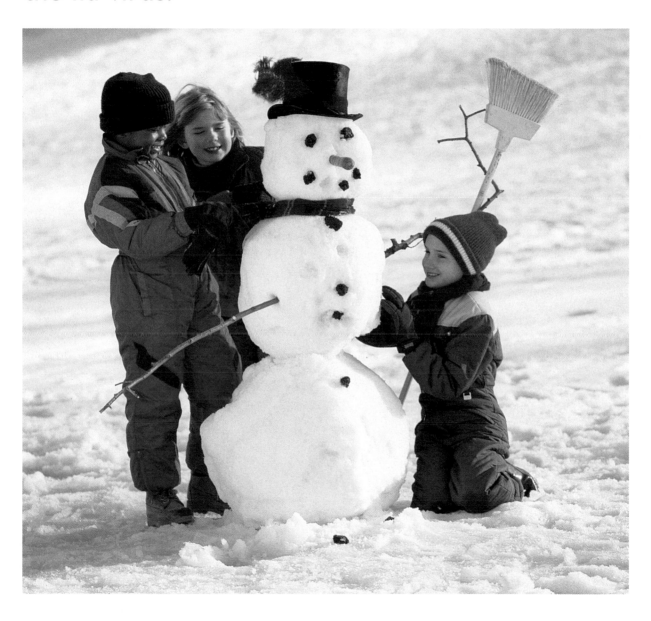

Flu Epidemics

Once in a while, many people get sick at the same time. This is called an **epidemic.** Many years ago, there was a very bad flu epidemic.

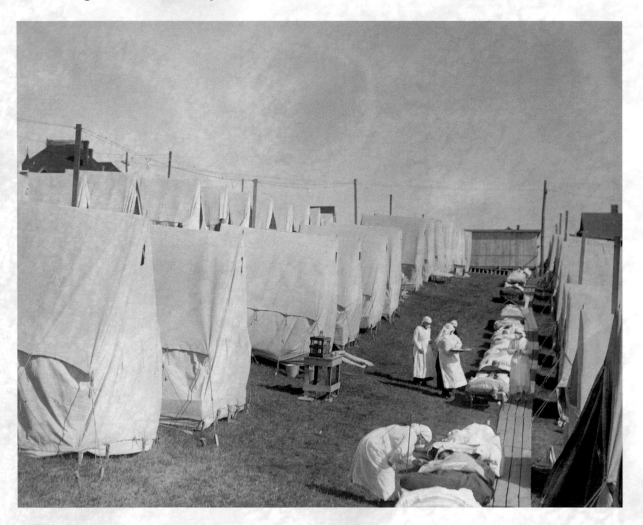

To keep from catching this flu, people wore masks over their noses and mouths. They hoped this would keep them from catching this terrible flu.

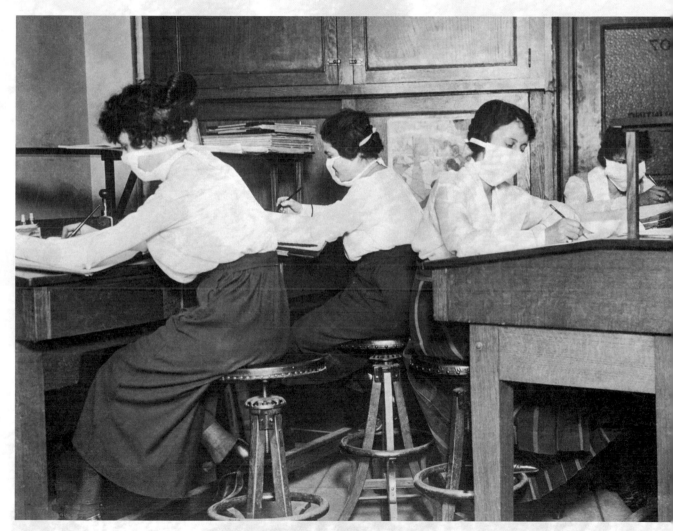

Staying Healthy

During flu season, try to stay away from crowded places. The more people you are near, the more likely you are to breathe in the flu **virus.**

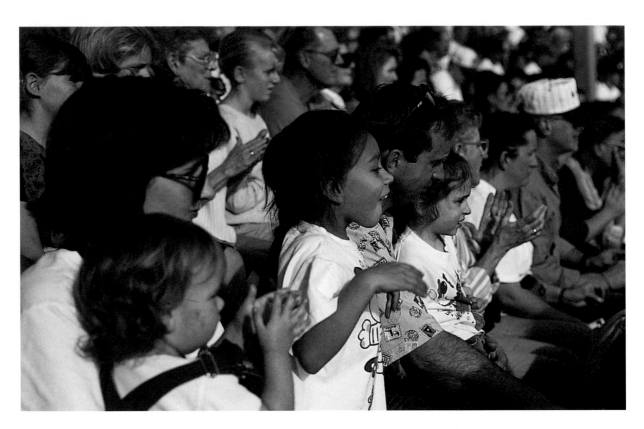

Also be sure to wash your hands often and keep them away from your nose and mouth. Eating right and getting enough sleep will also help keep your body strong and healthy.

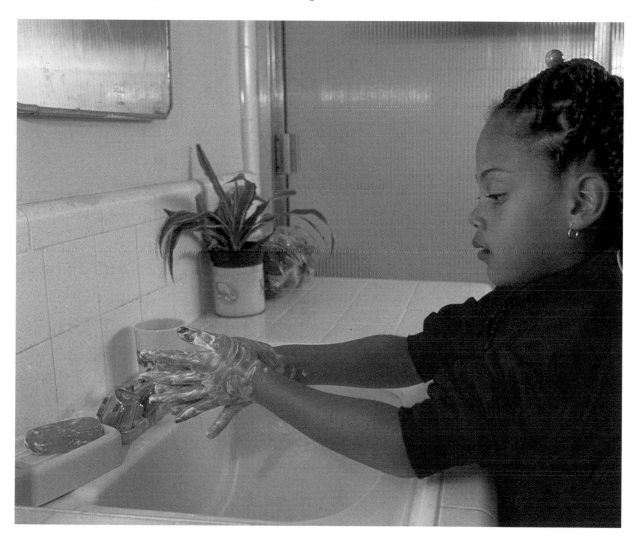

Think about It!

Carlos has flu. He has a **fever.** His head and his body hurt. What can his father do to help Carlos feel better?*

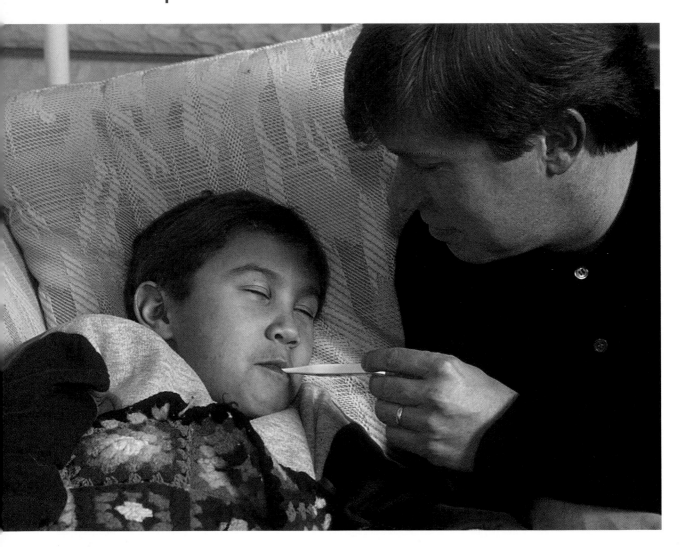

Mike's sister has flu. What can Mike do to keep from catching flu?*

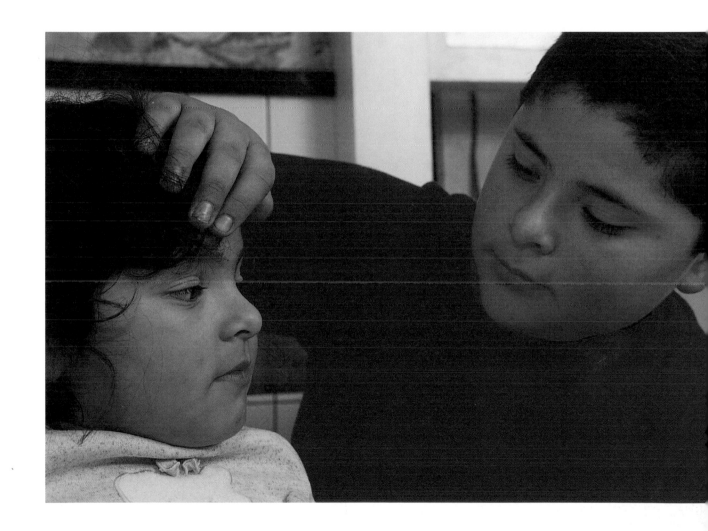

*Read page 30 to find out.

Answers

Page 28

Carlos's dad can give him some **pain relievers.** This will help make Carlos's head and body hurt less. The pain relievers will also make his **fever** go down.

Page 29

Mike should try to stay away from his sister. If he has to be near her, he should be sure to wash his hands often.

Stay Healthy and Safe!

1. Always tell an adult if you feel sick or think there is something wrong with you.

2. Never take any medicine unless it is given to you by an adult you trust.

3. Remember, the best way to stay healthy and safe is to eat good food, drink lots of water, keep clean, exercise, and get lots of sleep.

Glossary

epidemic   when many people have the same sickness at the same time

fever   when the temperature of your body becomes hotter than normal

germ   tiny thing that can make you ill if it gets in your body

immunity   protection from getting an illness

infection   illness caused by germs that can spread from one person to another

infectious   can be passed from one person to another and can make you sick

lung   part of your body inside your chest that helps you breathe. People have two lungs.

microscope   machine that makes very small things look big enough to see

mucous membrane   sticky lining in the nose and throat

pain reliever   medicine that gets rid of pain

pneumonia   type of dangerous lung infection

temperature   measure of how hot or cold something is

vaccine   shot that keeps people from getting a sickness

virus   tiny germ that can make you sick if it gets inside your body

Index

More Books to Read

Hundley, David H. *Viruses*. Vero Beach, Fla.: Rourke Press, 1998.

Royston, Angela. *Clean and Healthy*. Chicago: Heinemann Library, 1999.

Weitzman, Elizabeth. *Let's Talk about Having the Flu*. New York: Rosen Publishing Group, 1997.